Table Of Contents

I. Introduction

Overview of Diet and Nutrition

Diet refers to the types of food a person eats on a regular basis and the way they consume them. Nutrition, on the other hand, is the study of how food affects the body and how the body uses the food to maintain good health.

Importance of a Healthy Diet

A healthy diet is essential for overall well-being and longevity. It can reduce the risk of chronic diseases such as heart disease, obesity, and type 2 diabetes. A well-balanced diet can also improve mental health and mood, enhance physical performance, and boost the immune system.

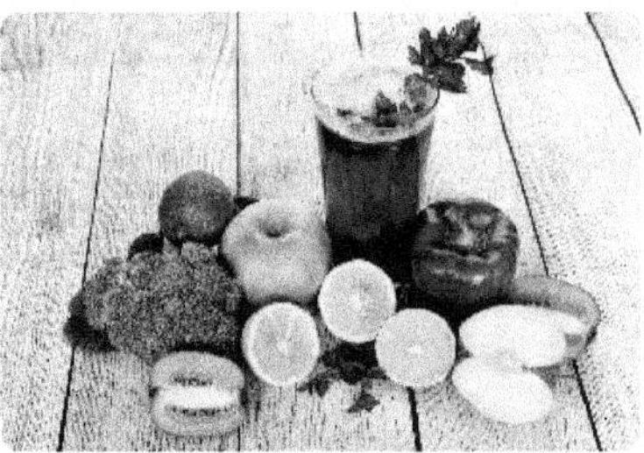

This guide aims to provide a comprehensive overview of diet and nutrition for beginners. It covers the basics of nutrition, recommended food groups, what to avoid, meal planning, and preparation, special dietary needs, and supplements. The guide is designed to help individuals make informed choices about their food and nutrition and to adopt a healthy eating lifestyle.

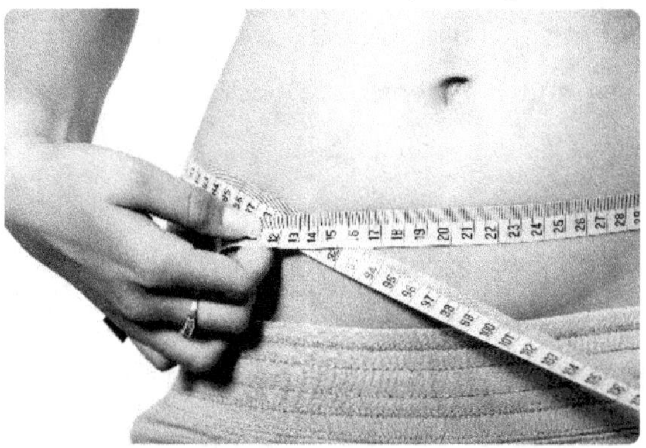

This guide is intended for individuals who are new to diet and nutrition and looking to improve their overall health and well-being. Whether you are seeking to lose weight, build muscle, or simply maintain a healthy lifestyle, this guide provides the necessary information and practical tips to help you achieve your goals.

II. Understanding Basic Nutrition

Macronutrients

Proteins : Essential building blocks of the body and essential for cell repair, growth, and maintenance. Good sources of protein include meat, fish, eggs, dairy products, beans, and legumes.

Fats : An important energy source and essential for the absorption of vitamins A, D, E, and K. Good sources of healthy fats include nuts, seeds, avocados, olive oil, and fatty fish.

Carbohydrates : The primarysource of energy for the body. Good sources of carbohydrates include fruits, vegetables, grains, and legumes.

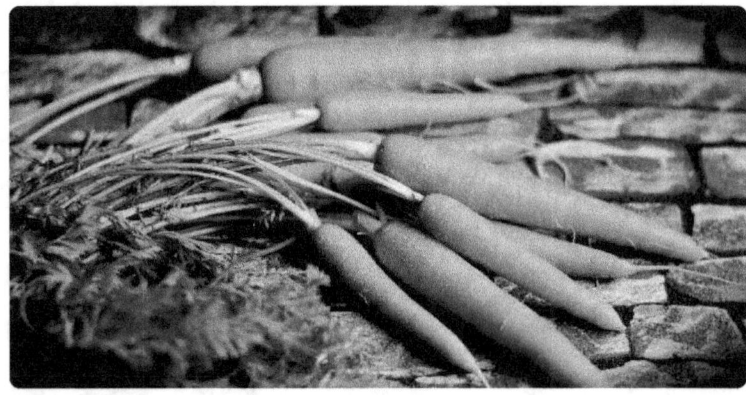

Micronutrients

Vitamins : Essential for various functions in the body, such as maintaining a healthy immune system, protecting the eyes, and helping with blood clotting. Good sources of vitamins include fruits, vegetables, dairy products, and fortified cereals.

Minerals : Essential for various functions in the body, such as maintaining a healthy heart, bones, and teeth. Good sources of minerals include leafy greens, nuts, seeds, dairy products, and seafood.

Water and Fiber

Water : Essential for the proper functioning of the body and helps regulate body temperature, transport nutrients, and eliminate waste.

Fiber : Essential for maintaining a healthy digestive system and reducing the risk of heart disease and type 2 diabetes. Good sources of fiber include fruits, vegetables, whole grains, and legumes.

Energy Balance and Weight Management

Energy balance refers to the balance between the calories consumed and the calories burned. To maintain a healthy weight, it is important to find a balance between the calories consumed and the calories burned through physical activity. Overconsumption of calories and lack of physical activity can lead to weight gain, while undereating and over-exercising can lead to weight loss.

Daily Requirements

The daily requirement of macronutrients and micronutrients varies depending on age, gender, and physical activity levels. It is important to consult a healthcare professional or a registered dietitian to determine your individual needs.

III. Recommended Food Groups

Fruits and Vegetables

Fruits and vegetables are essential sources of vitamins, minerals, and fiber. It is recommended to consume a variety of colorful fruits and vegetables to ensure adequate intake of all essential nutrients. Aim to consume at least 5 servings of fruits and vegetables per day, with at least one serving of dark green leafy vegetables.

Grains and Legumes

Grains and legumes provide carbohydrates, fiber, and some protein. It is recommended to choose whole grain options, such as whole 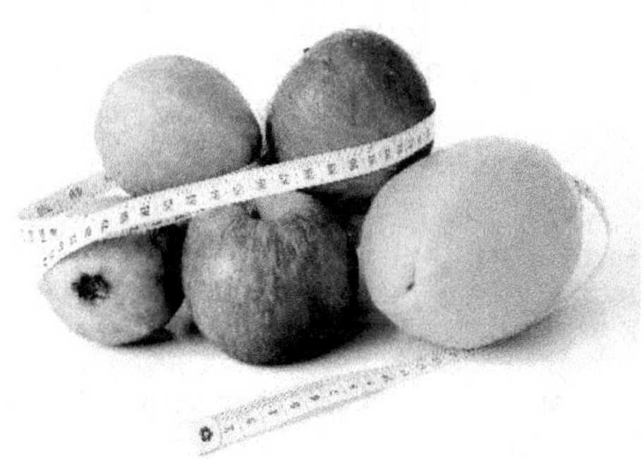 wheat bread, brown rice, and whole grain pasta, instead of refined grains. Legumes, such as beans, lentils, and chickpeas, are also good sources of protein and fiber.

Dairy and Dairy Alternatives

Dairy products provide calcium, which is essential for strong bones, and other vitamins and minerals. For those who are lactose intolerant or have other dietary restrictions, dairy alternatives, such as soy milk, almond milk, and coconut milk, are available. It is important to choose options that are fortified with calcium and other essential nutrients.

Meat and Protein Alternatives

Meat provides protein, iron, and other essential nutrients. It is recommended to choose lean cuts of meat, such as poultry and fish, and to limit the intake of red and processed meats. For those who follow a vegetarian or vegan diet, protein alternatives, such as tofu, tempeh, and lentils, are available.

Fats and Oils

Fats and oils are essential for the absorption of vitamins and for overall health. It is recommended to choose healthy fats, such as olive oil, nuts, and avocados, instead of unhealthy fats, such as trans and saturated fats. It is important to limit the intake of unhealthy fats, as they can increase the risk of heart disease and other chronic conditions.

Sweet Treats and Beverages

Sweet treats and beverages, such as candy, cake, and soda, are sources of added sugars and should be consumed in moderation. It is recommended to choose healthier options, such as fruit, herbal tea, and water, as a source of hydration and sweet flavor. It is important to be mindful of the added sugars in beverages, as they can contribute to weight gain and other health problems.

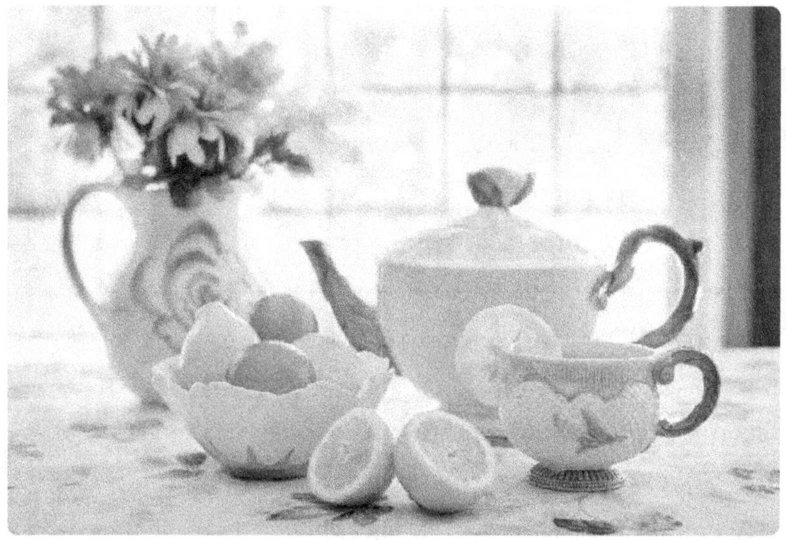

IV. What to Avoid

Processed foods, such as packaged snacks, convenience meals, and fried foods, are often high in unhealthy fats, added sugars, and preservatives. They can contribute to weight gain, poor nutrition, and increased risk of chronic diseases. It is recommended to limit the consumption of processed foods and choose whole, unprocessed foods instead.

Added sugars, such as those found in soda, candy, and sweetened beverages, can contribute to weight gain, poor nutrition, and increased risk of chronic diseases, such as type 2 diabetes and heart disease. It is recommended to limit the intake of added sugars and choose natural sources of sweetness, such as fruit.

Sodium, found in processed and packaged foods, can contribute to high blood pressure and increased risk of heart disease. It is recommended to limit the intake of sodium and choose low-sodium options, such as fresh fruits and vegetables, whole grains, and lean protein sources.

Saturated and trans fats, found in animal products and processed foods, can increase the risk of heart disease and other chronic conditions. It is recommended to limit the intake of saturated and trans fats and choose healthy fats, such as olive oil, nuts, and avocados.

Alcohol is a source of empty calories and can contribute to weight gain and poor nutrition. It is also associated with increased risk of chronic diseases, such as liver disease and certain types of cancer. It is recommended to limit the intake of alcohol and choose water, herbal tea, and other low-calorie beverages instead.

Caffeine, found in coffee, tea, and energy drinks, can disrupt sleep, increase anxiety, and cause other health problems. It is recommended to limit the intake of caffeine and choose decaffeinated options or herbal tea instead. It is important to be mindful of the amount of caffeine consumed and its effects on individual health.

V. Meal Planning and Preparation

Importance of Meal Planning

Meal planning can help ensure a balanced and nutritious diet, reduce food waste, and save time and money. It involves creating a plan for weekly meals, snacks, and grocery shopping.

Steps for Effective Meal Planning

Assess personal nutrition needs and goals.

Create a weekly menu, taking into consideration food preferences, dietary restrictions, and schedule.

Make a grocery list based on the weekly menu and stick to it while shopping.

Prepare and store meals ahead of time, as needed.

Keep healthy snacks on hand for when hunger strikes.

Advantages of Meal Planning and Preparation

Helps achieve and maintain a balanced and nutritious diet

Saves time and money

Reduces food waste

Increases food variety and reduces the risk of boredom with meals

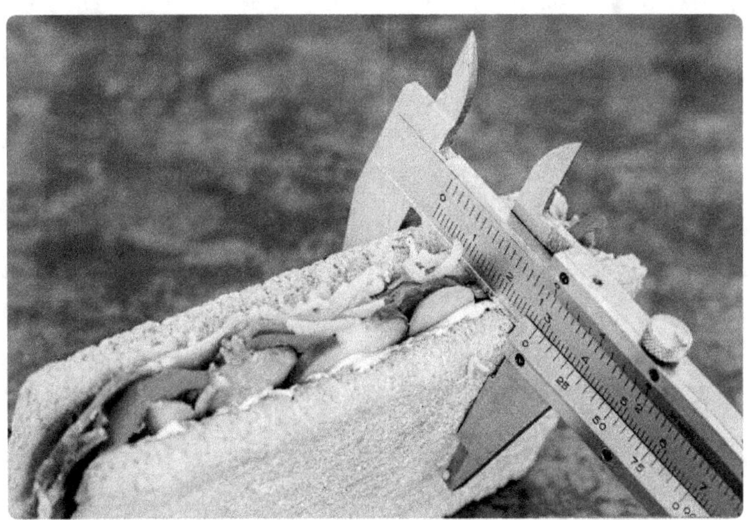

Tips for Meal Preparation

Use a slow cooker or pressure cooker to prepare meals ahead of time.

Freeze meals in single portions for easy grab-and-go options.

Prepare simple, quick meals, such as salads, stir-fries, and sandwiches, for busy nights.

Use leftovers for lunch the next day or for future meals.

Get creative with meal preparation, trying new recipes and ingredients.

Meal planning and preparation are important steps in maintaining a balanced and nutritious diet. By taking the time to plan and prepare meals, individuals can ensure that they are consuming the essential nutrients needed for good health.

VI. Special Dietary Needs

Vegetarian and Vegan Diets

Vegetarian diets exclude meat and fish, while vegan diets exclude all animal products, including eggs and dairy.

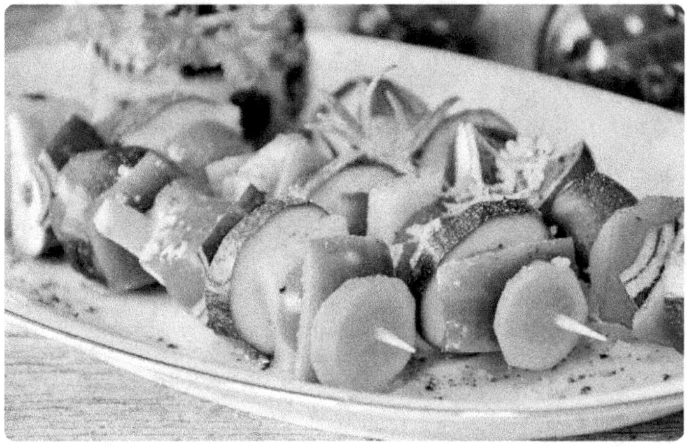

A well-planned vegetarian or vegan diet can provide all the necessary nutrients for good health, but it is important to pay attention to key nutrients, such as protein, iron, calcium, and vitamin B12.

Recommendations for a healthy vegetarian or vegan diet include incorporating a variety of plant-based protein sources, such as legumes, nuts, and tofu, and taking a vitamin B12 supplement, if needed.

Gluten-Free Diet

A gluten-free diet is necessary for individuals with celiac disease or non-celiac gluten sensitivity. Gluten is a protein found in wheat, barley, and rye.

A gluten-free diet requires avoiding these grains and choosing alternative grains, such as quinoa, rice, and corn. It is important to read food labels carefully and to choose naturally gluten-free foods, such as fruits and vegetables, in addition to gluten-free grains.

Low-FODMAP Diet

A low-FODMAP diet is designed to help individuals with irritable bowel syndrome (IBS) manage their symptoms.

FODMAPs are short-chain carbohydrates that can cause digestive discomfort for some individuals.

A low-FODMAP diet involves avoiding foods high in FODMAPs, such as certain fruits, vegetables, grains, and dairy products, and choosing low-FODMAP alternatives. It is important to work with a healthcare provider and a registered dietitian to ensure that all necessary nutrients are being consumed while following a low-FODMAP diet.

Other Special Dietary Needs

Other special dietary needs, such as kosher, halal, and low-sodium diets, require following specific guidelines and avoiding certain foods.

It is important to work with a healthcare provider and a registered dietitian to ensure that all necessary nutrients are being consumed while following a special diet.

Special dietary needs, such as vegetarian and vegan diets, gluten-free diets, and low-FODMAP diets, require careful planning and attention to key nutrients. By working with a healthcare provider and a registered dietitian, individuals with special dietary needs can ensure that they are consuming a balanced and nutritious diet.

VII. Supplements

Supplements are products taken orally to add nutrients to the diet that may be missing or in insufficient quantities. They come in a variety of forms, including pills, capsules, powders, and liquids.

When to Consider Supplements :

Supplements may be necessary for individuals with specific health conditions, such as anemia or osteoporosis, or for those following special diets, such as vegetarian or vegan diets. They may also be recommended for individuals who are unable to consume sufficient amounts of certain nutrients from food sources. It is important to speak with a healthcare provider or a registered dietitian before starting any supplement regimen.

Types of Supplements

Multivitamin and mineral supplements: provide a combination of essential vitamins and minerals in one pill. Vitamin and mineral supplements: individual vitamins and minerals, such as vitamin C and iron, can be taken separately to address specific deficiencies. Herb and botanical supplements: plants and plant extracts, such as ginkgo biloba and echinacea, used for their potential health benefits. Protein supplements: provide additional protein to the diet, especially for individuals who are vegetarian or vegan.

Considerations for Taking Supplements :

Quality control : look for supplements that have been third-party tested for purity and potency.

Dosage : follow recommended dosages on the label and speak with a healthcare provider or registered dietitian about appropriate amounts for specific health conditions or goals.

Interactions : some supplements may interact with prescription medications or other supplements, so it is important to speak with a healthcare provider before starting any new supplement regimen.

IX. Conclusion

A. Summary of Key Points :

In this book, we have discussed the basics of diet and nutrition, including the recommended food groups, what to avoid, and meal planning and preparation. We also explored the role of supplements, special dietary needs, and strategies for staying on track with a healthier diet.

B. Importance of a Balanced Diet :

A balanced diet, including a variety of nutrient-dense foods from all food groups, is essential for overall health and wellness. By making small changes, such as incorporating more fruits and vegetables into meals, reducing sugar consumption, and choosing whole grains, individuals can improve their diet and enhance their health.

C. Consultation with a Healthcare Professional :

It is important to consult with a healthcare professional or a registered dietitian to determine individual nutritional needs and to address any specific health concerns. Healthcare professionals can provide personalized recommendations and support for making healthy changes to the diet.

D. Emphasizing Whole Foods :

Emphasizing whole, unprocessed foods, such as fruits, vegetables, whole grains, lean proteins, and healthy fats, is the foundation of a healthy diet.

Minimizing the consumption of processed, high-sugar, and high-fat foods can also help individuals improve their diet and enhance their health.

E. Final Thoughts :

A healthy diet plays a critical role in overall health and wellness. By making informed choices about food and nutrition, individuals can take control of their health and improve their quality of life. By following the guidelines outlined in this ebook, individuals can make sustainable changes to their diet and achieve their goals for improved health and wellness.

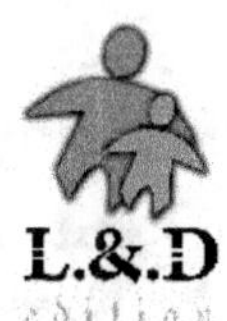

L.&.D
edition

L.&.D edition

2023

History Of Spirituality

Civilizations

Religions

Cultures & Societies

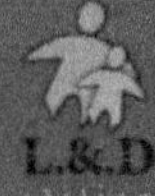

Table Of Contents

Spirituality can be defined as the personal and subjective experience of connecting with the divine or a higher power, or with a sense of purpose and meaning beyond the material world. It can be expressed through religious or non-religious beliefs, practices, and rituals.

Spirituality encompasses a wide range of beliefs, values, and experiences that provide individuals with a sense of peace, happiness, and fulfillment. It can be a source of comfort, inspiration, and guidance in times of need, and can help to bring meaning and purpose to one's life.

The study of spirituality is crucial for understanding the impact that it has had on human history, cultures, and societies. It sheds light on the beliefs, values, and practices that have shaped the way people think, act, and interact with one another.

Spirituality has played a significant role in shaping the development of human civilization, from shaping the ways people perceive the world and their place within it, to influencing political, social, and economic structures. The study of spirituality also provides insight into the evolution of human thought, beliefs, and practices over time.